This book is dedicated to the memory of my Mother, whose keen intellect, courage and compassion continue to inspire me. Even as her dementia worsened, my Mother retained her deep love for her family, especially her grandchildren. She would have wanted this story to be told, to help families with children understand this disease and to remember that even unspoken love is still love.

When My Grammy Forgets, I Remember: A Child's Perspective on Dementia

Published by Baypointe Publishers

Editor@BaypointePublishers.com

ISBN 978-0-9916236-0-0   Paperback

ISBN 978-0-9916236-1-7   E-Book

Library of Congress Control Number: 2014919481

Summary:

Every day when Elise gets off the school bus, her Grammy is waiting for her, ready to make a cheese sandwich and share knock-knock jokes. Then Grammy begins to lose her keys and gets lost coming home. Elise is worried. Mom explains in a simple manner that Grammy has dementia. Elise realizes that although Grammy's illness has altered their relationship, their love for each other continues.

Interest age level: 5 and up.

Children's Books > Family Life > Growing up & Facts of Life > Difficult Discussions > Illness

When My Grammy Forgets, I Remember:
A Child's Perspective on Dementia

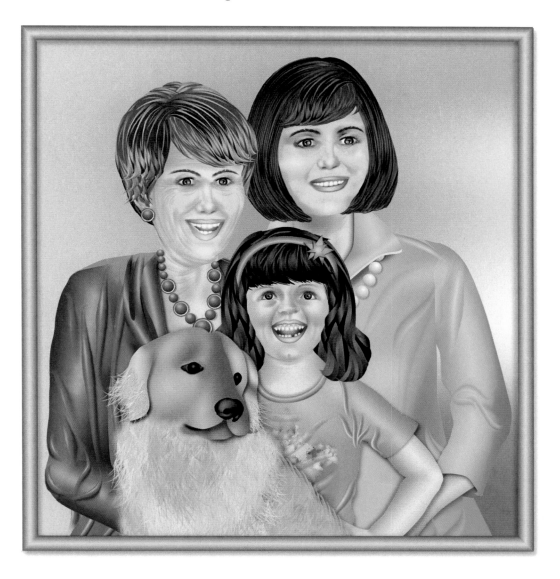

Written by Toby Haberkorn
Illustrations by Heather Varkarotas

I love my Grammy!

Grammy smells like roses and always gives me kisses.

She asks me about my school day

and listens to what I have to say.

My Grammy hugs me tight.

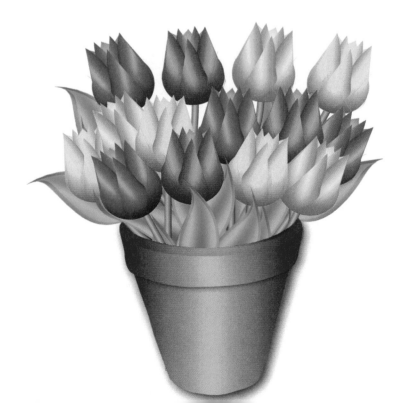

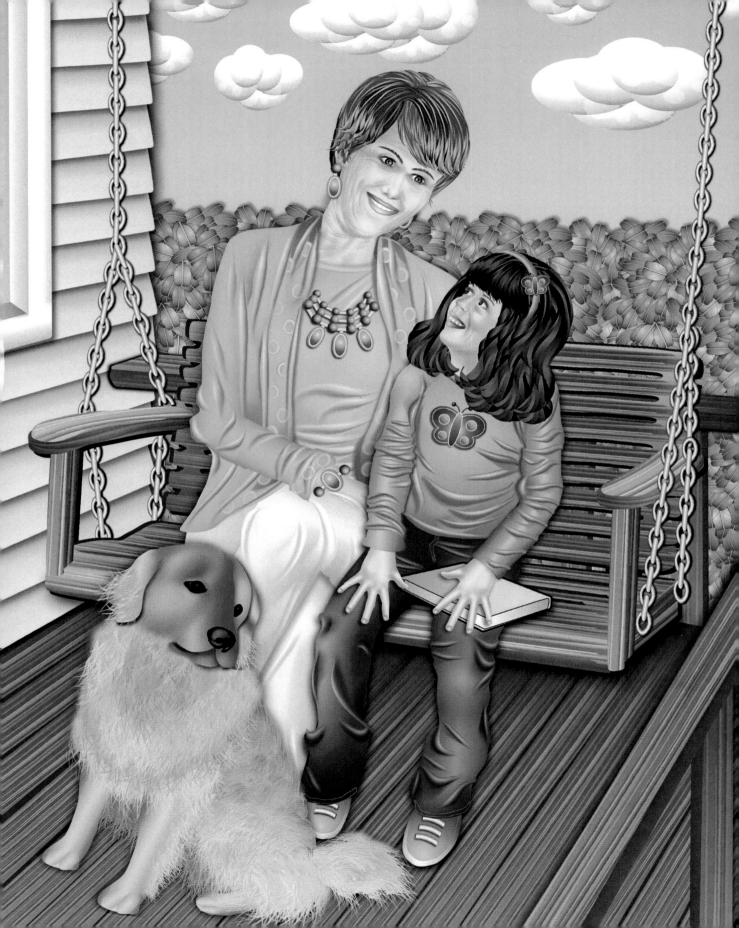

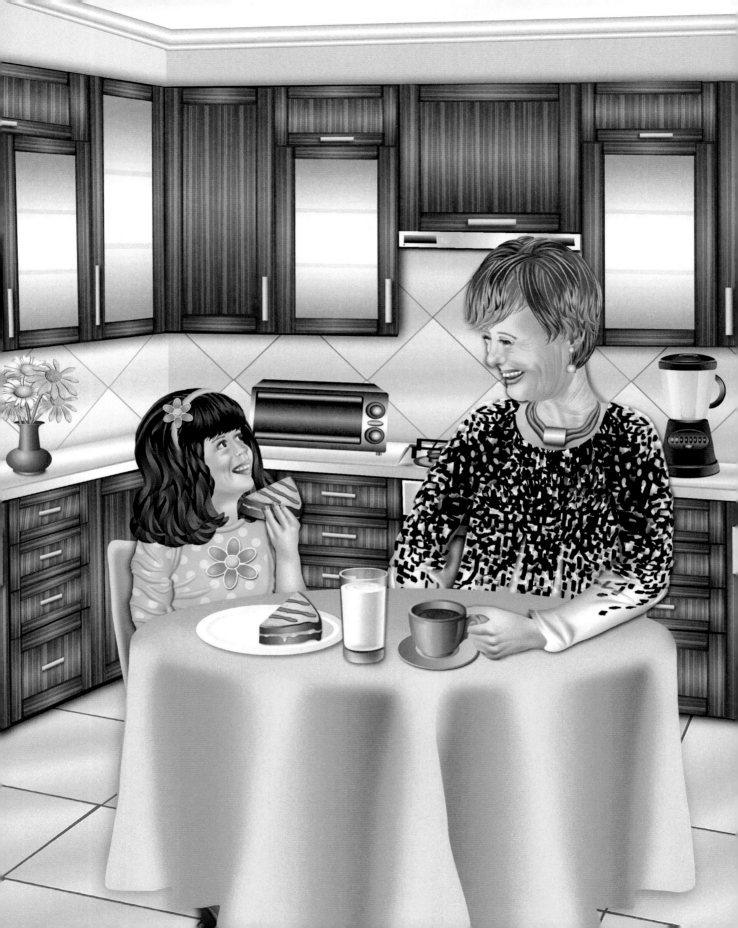

Grammy picks me up from school.

She makes me toasted cheese sandwiches for snacks.

Her sandwiches are better than yummy.

My Grammy hugs me tight.

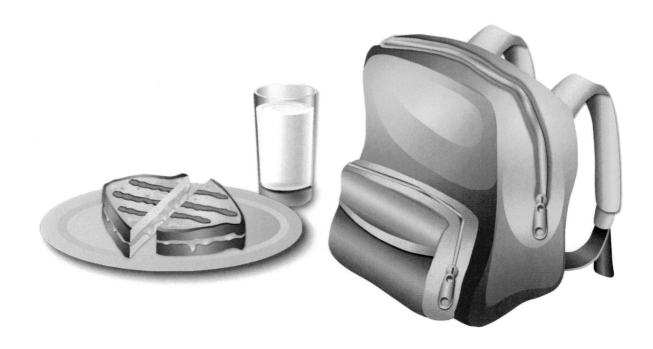

Grammy says she loves my dimples.

I tell Grammy I will iron her wrinkles away.

She laughs and they disappear.

My Grammy hugs me tight.

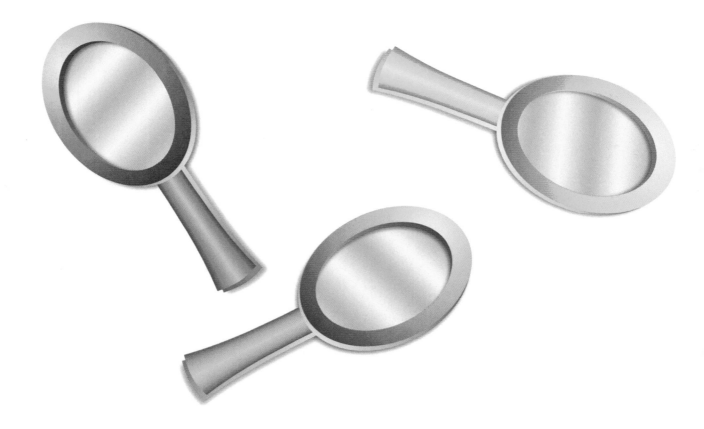

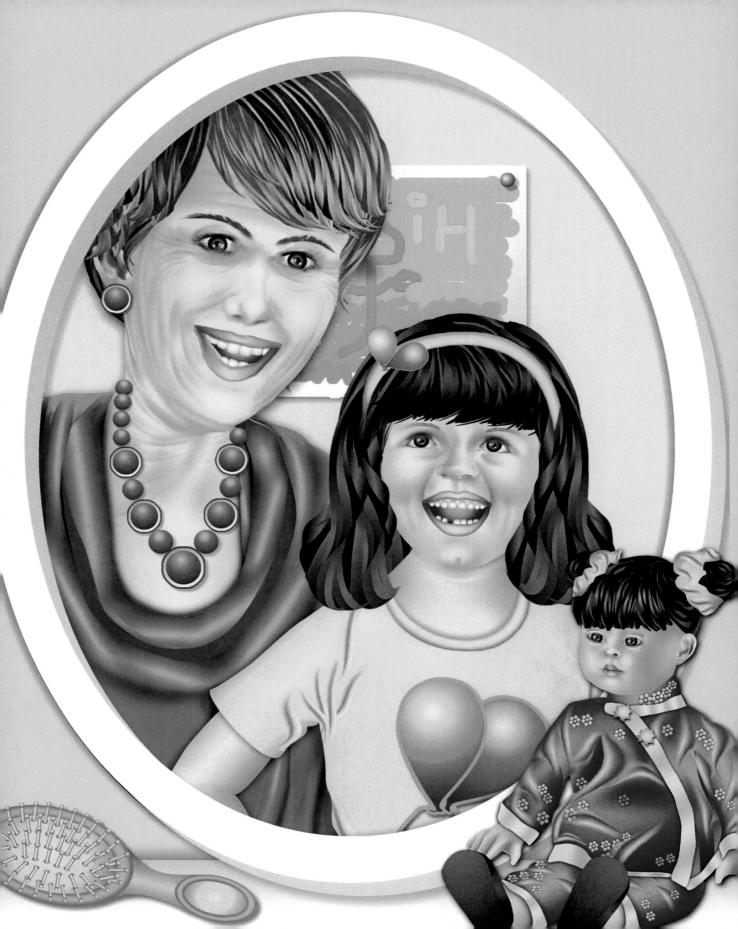

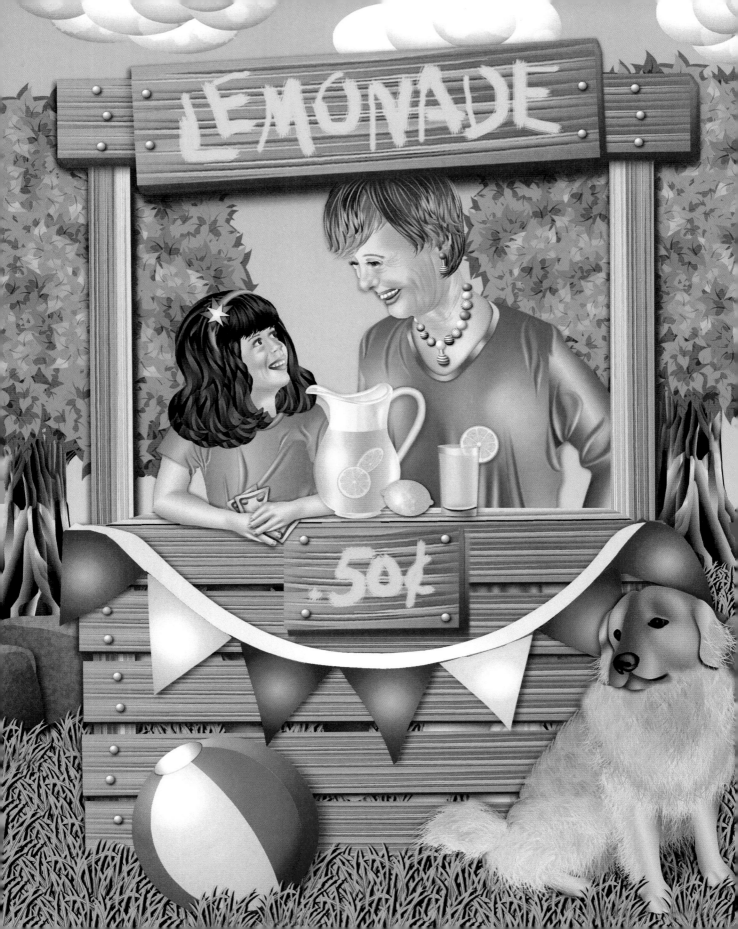

Grammy helps me squeeze lemons.

We count the money from my lemonade stand.

I have enough to buy a new book.

My Grammy hugs me tight.

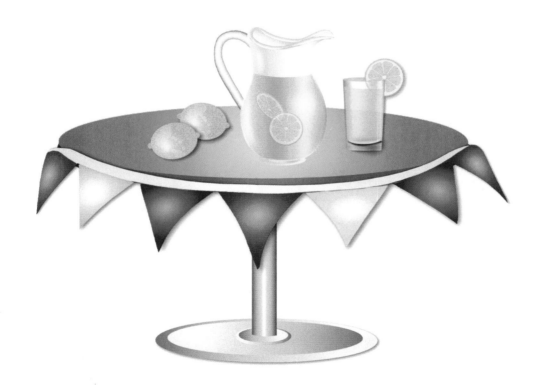

Grammy plays Bridge on Wednesdays.

I place the nuts, chocolates and hard candies on the table.

Grammy wins almost all her games.

My Grammy hugs me tight.

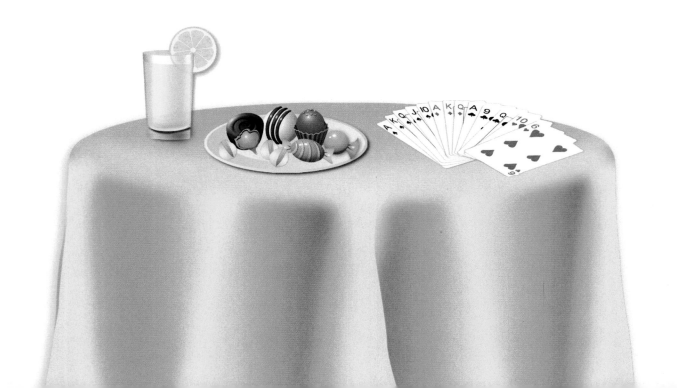

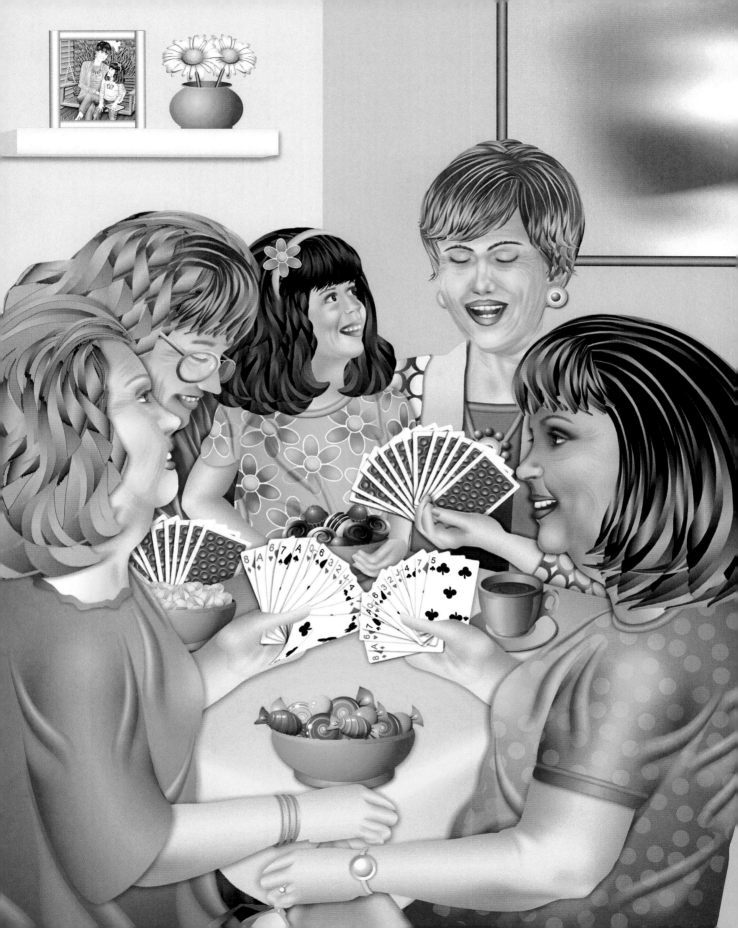

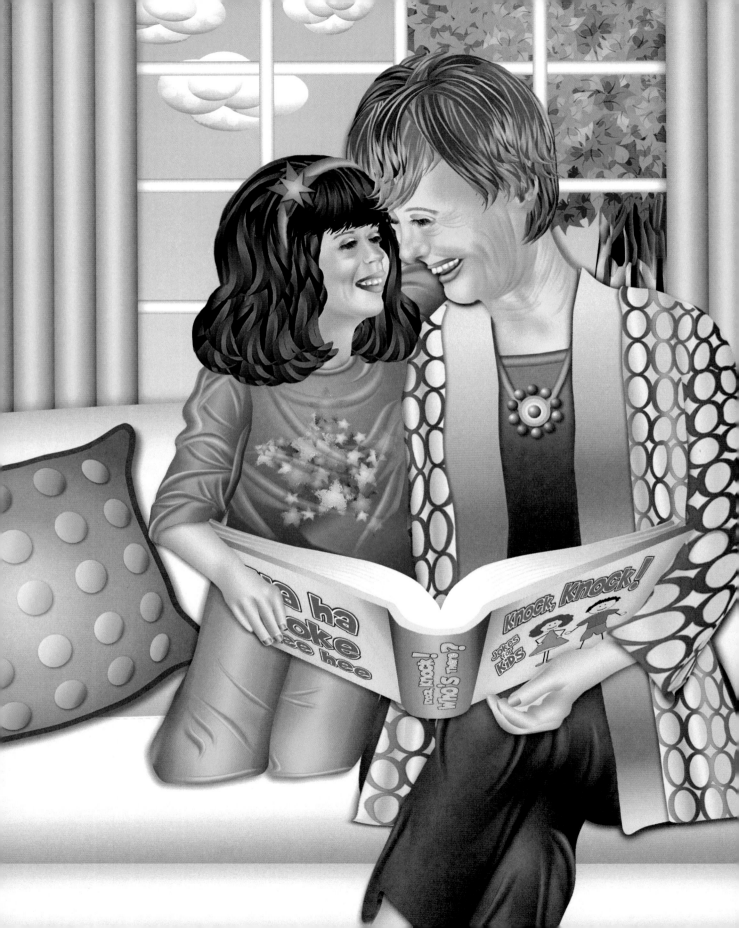

Grammy smiles all the time.

We tell each other knock-knock jokes.

My jokes are funnier than hers.

My Grammy hugs me tight.

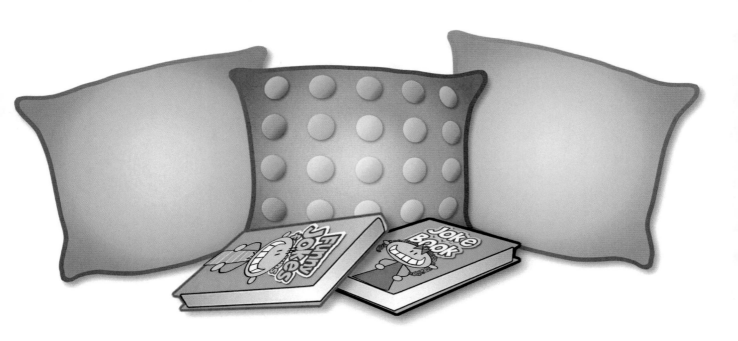

Grammy takes lots of trips to far away countries.

She brings me back dolls from many places.

Together we make up stories about them.

My Grammy hugs me tight.

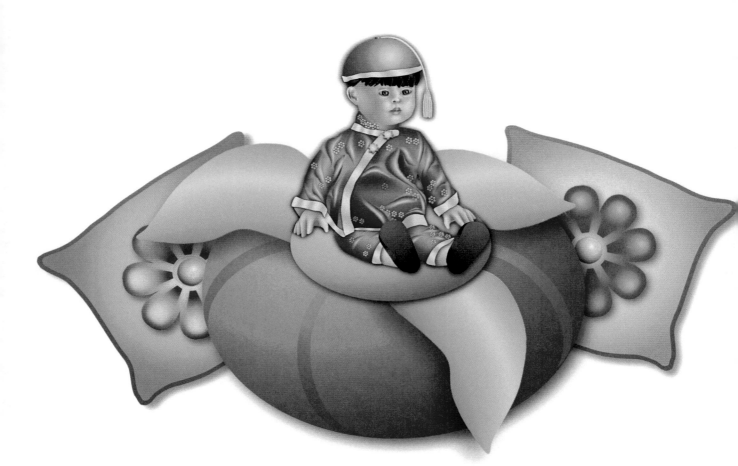

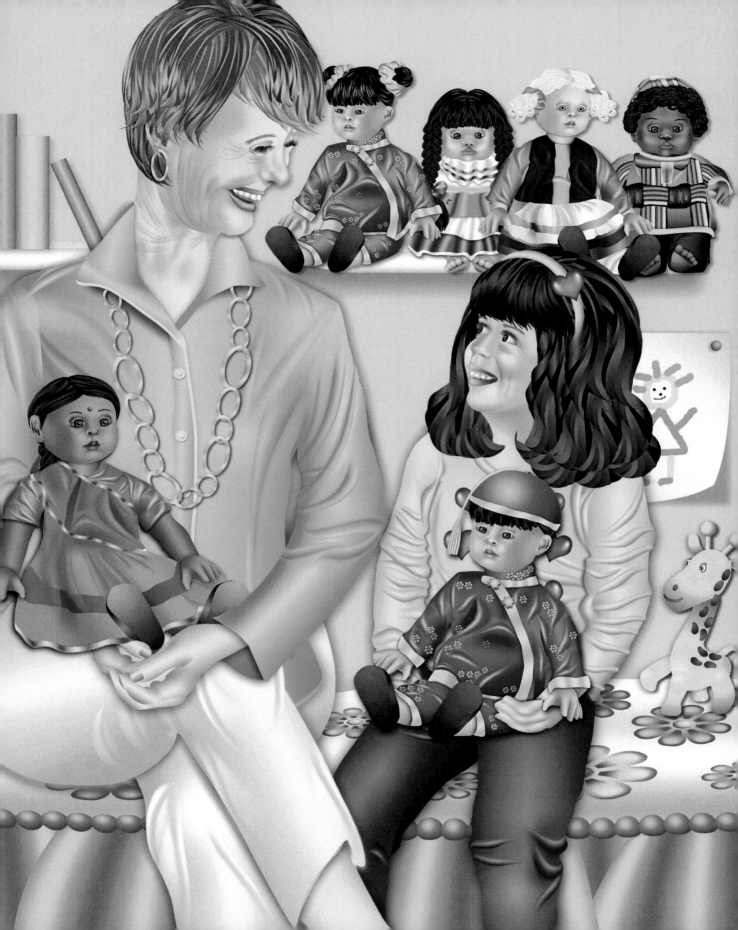

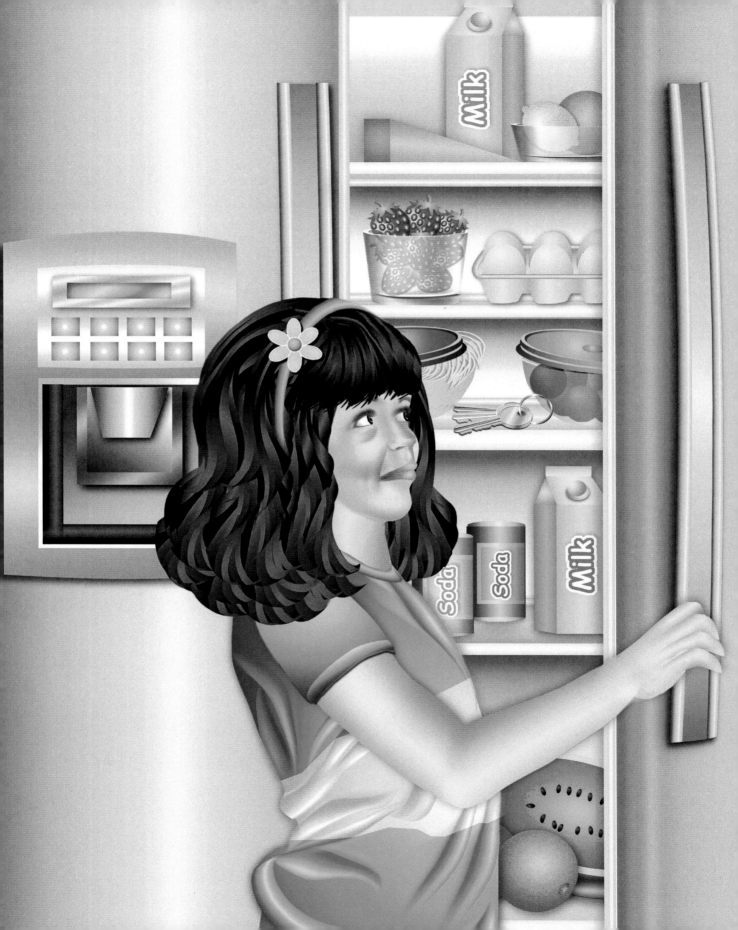

Grammy misplaces her keys.

Sometimes she puts them in the refrigerator.

I know where the spare key is hidden.

I hug my Grammy tight.

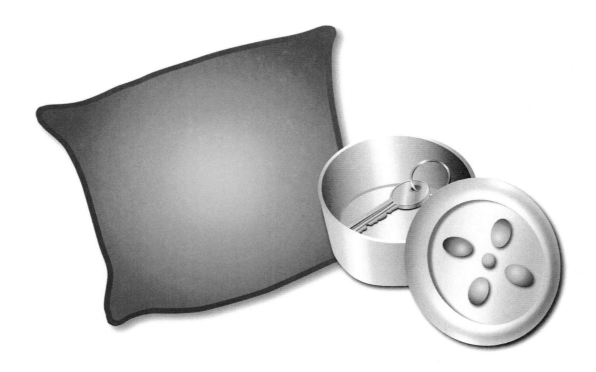

Grammy reads to me at bedtime.

She stares at the pages.

And sometimes forgets how to read.

"Grammy, you know these words," I say.

She shakes her head.

I hug my Grammy tight.

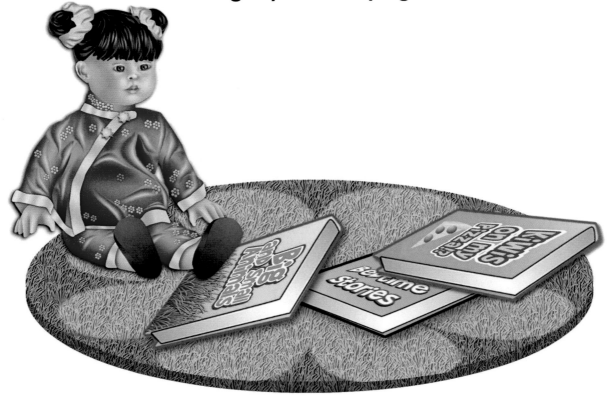

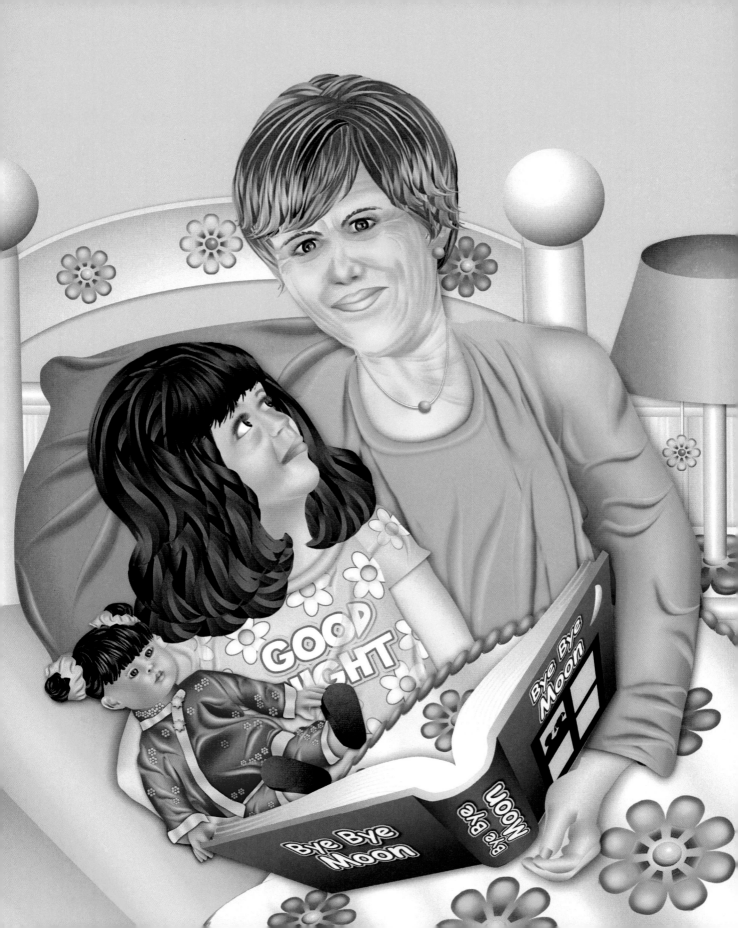

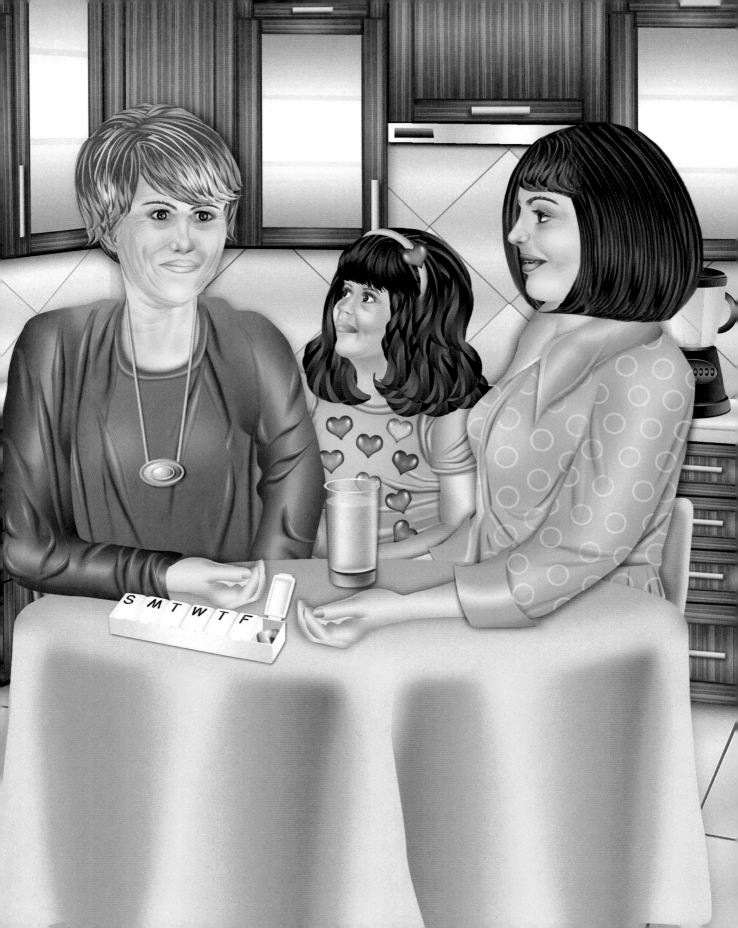

Grammy forgets to take her medicine.

Mom carefully puts her pills in special boxes.

I give Grammy a glass of water.

I hug my Grammy tight.

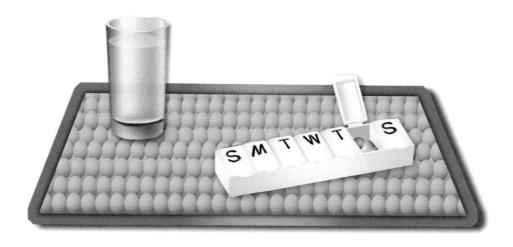

Grammy forgets what she is doing or where she is.

Mom now takes care of her.

"What's wrong with Grammy?" I worry.

Mom says Grammy's brain is not working properly.

"Does my Grammy still love me?" I ask.

"Yes, she will always love you."

My mommy hugs me tight.

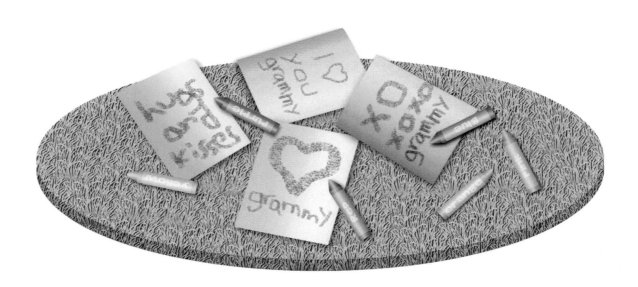

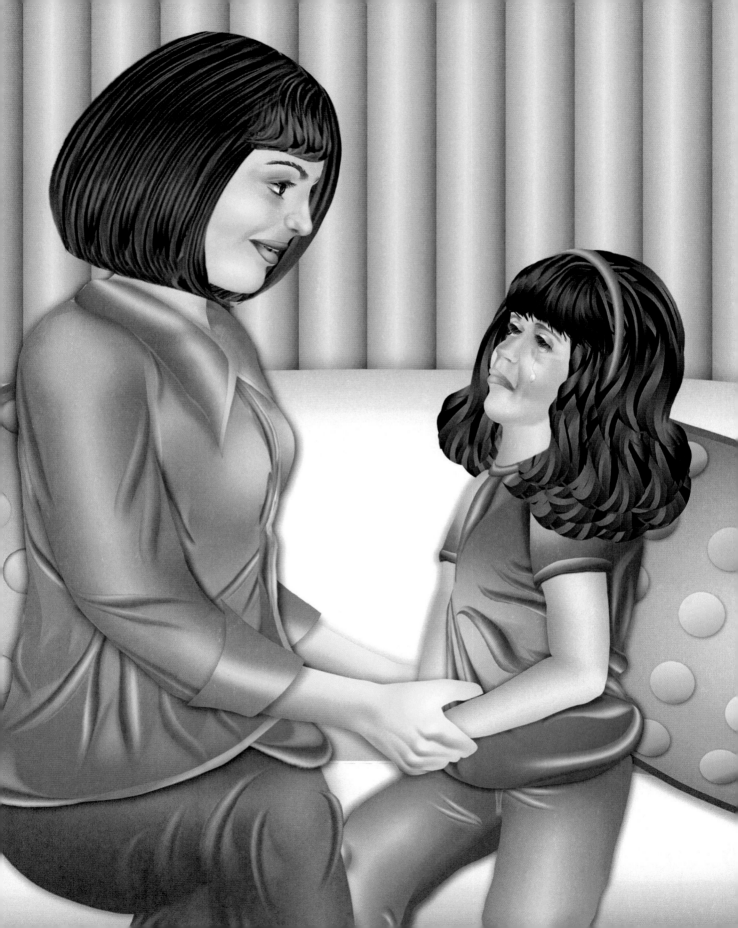

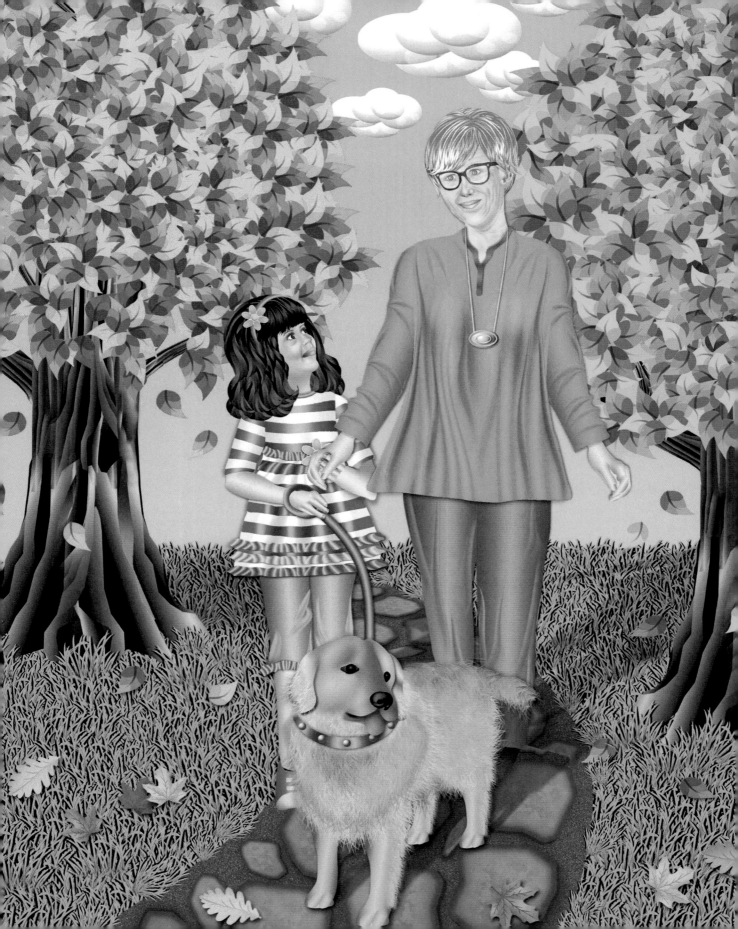

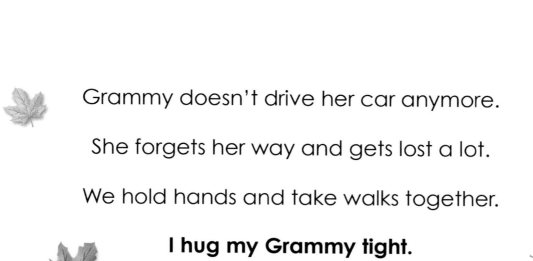

Grammy doesn't drive her car anymore.

She forgets her way and gets lost a lot.

We hold hands and take walks together.

I hug my Grammy tight.

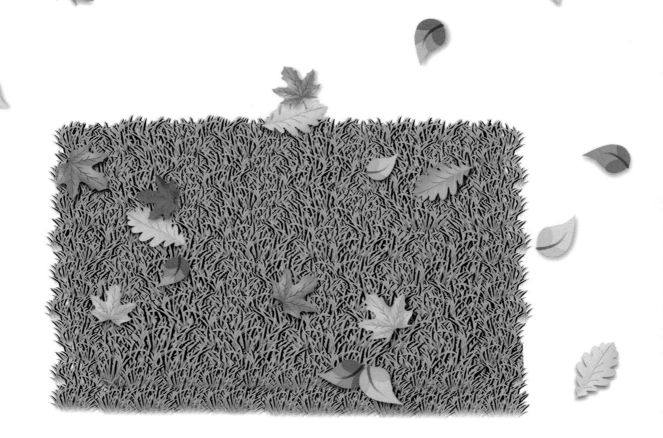

Grammy sometimes calls me Beth, my mom's name.

I don't mind so much anymore.

Grammy remembers my mom as a child.

I hug my Grammy tight.

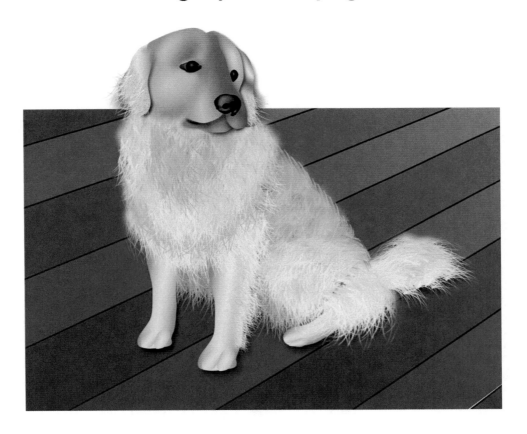

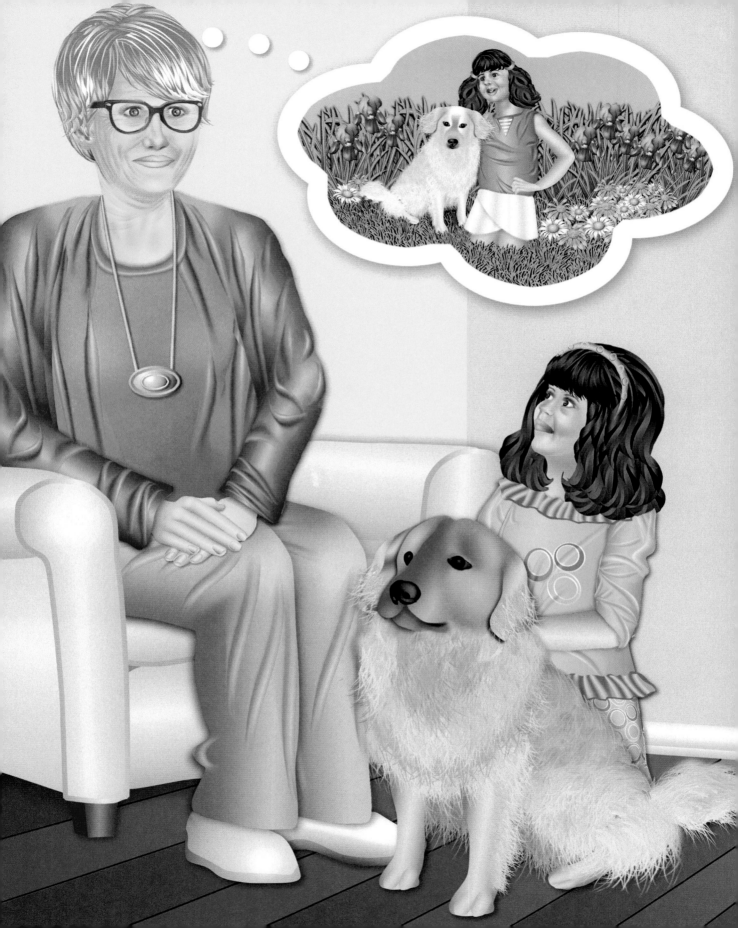

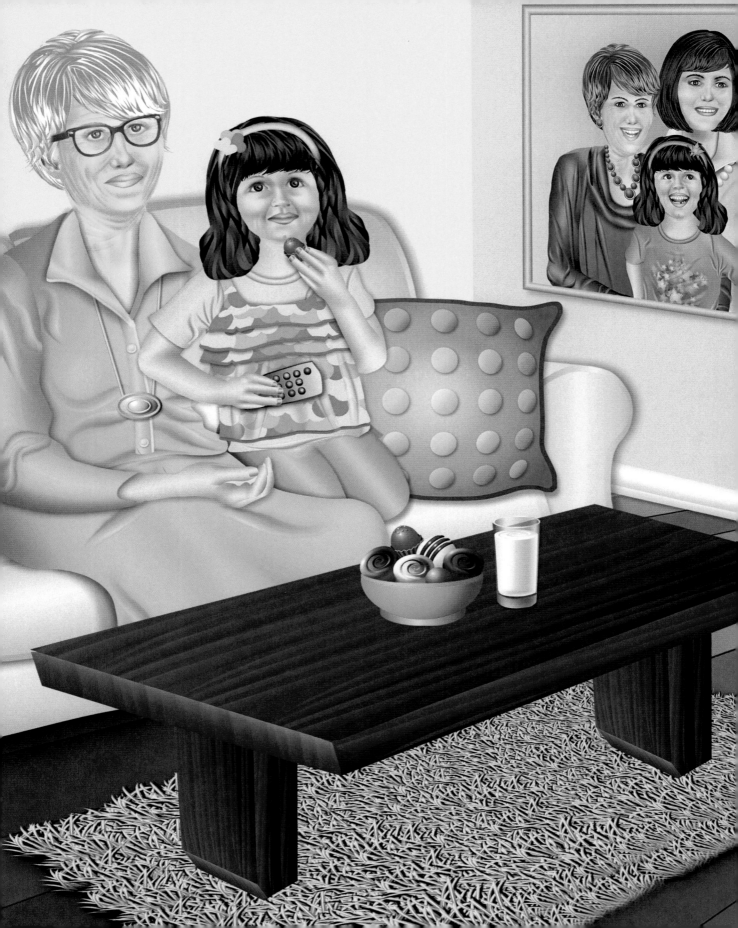

Grammy doesn't play cards with her friends anymore.

She forgets the rules.

We watch TV together and eat chocolates.

I hug my Grammy tight.

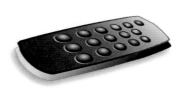

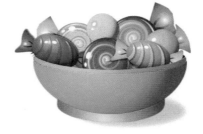

Grammy doesn't read anymore.

We sit on the sofa and I read to her.

Grammy sometimes turns the pages for me.

I hug my Grammy tight.

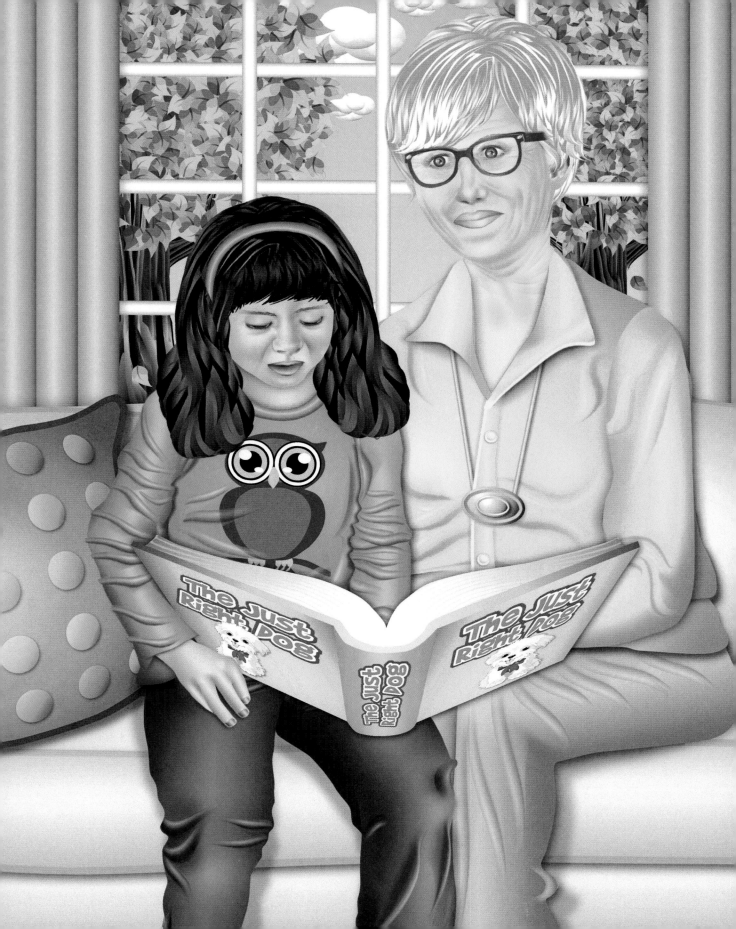

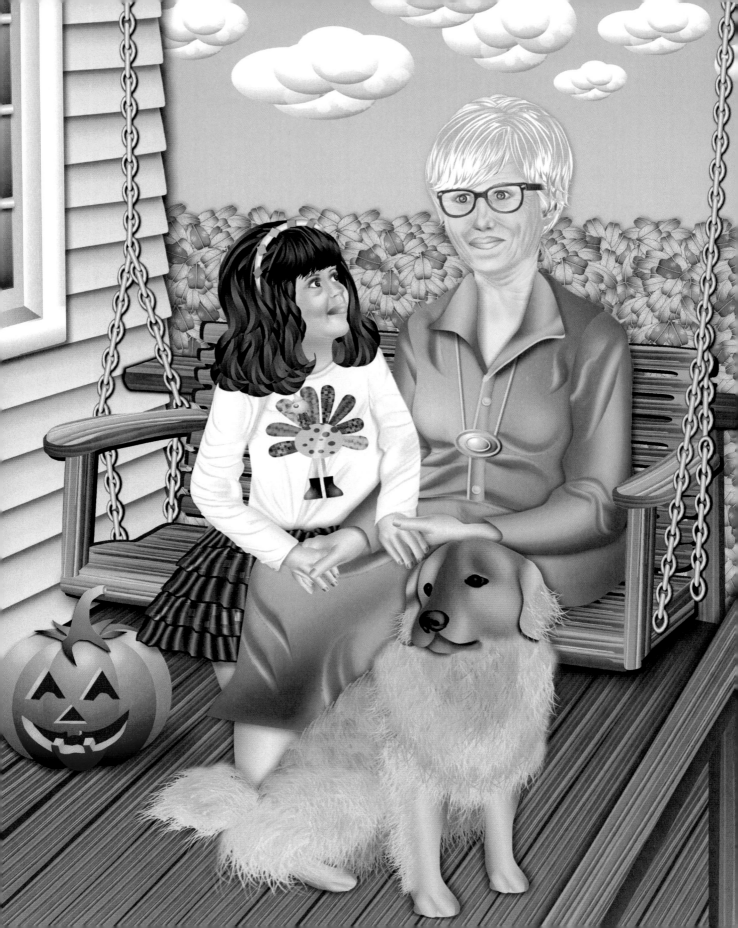

I feel sad.

I remember the way my Grammy used to be.

My jokes made her laugh.

She is different now, but I will always love her.

I know my Grammy loves me.

I hold her hand and hope she'll smile.

We hug each other tight.

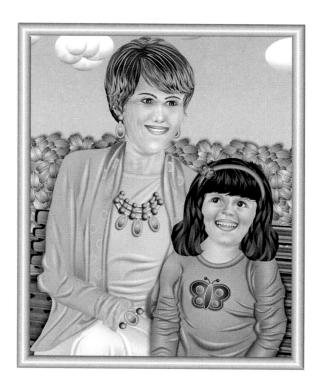

About the Author

Growing up in Cleveland, Ohio, Toby Haberkorn was a voracious reader. Later, as a young mother, she delighted in creating stories for her children. **When My Grammy Forgets, I Remember: A Child's Perspective on Dementia** was inspired by Toby's own family's experiences with her mother's dementia. Toby currently lives in Texas, with her family, where she is working on her next book. Her hope is that this book will raise awareness and help families and children better understand this debilitating disease.